MW00882298

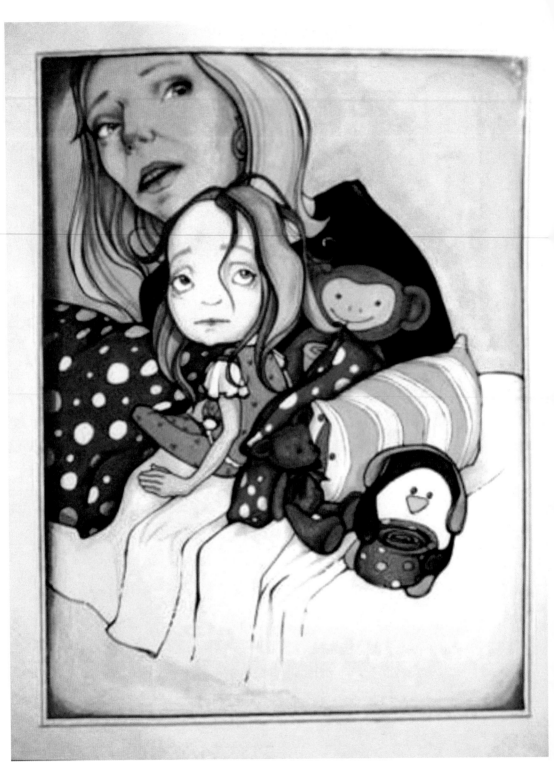

One morning I woke up and something different happened. I don't remember anything but my mom has never forgotten. She said I was asleep and all of a sudden, I was making strange noises and the left side of my face was moving funny. She was very scared and called for my older sister as she tried to wake me. She said when I finally opened my eyes; I was drooling heavily, looked scared and was very confused.

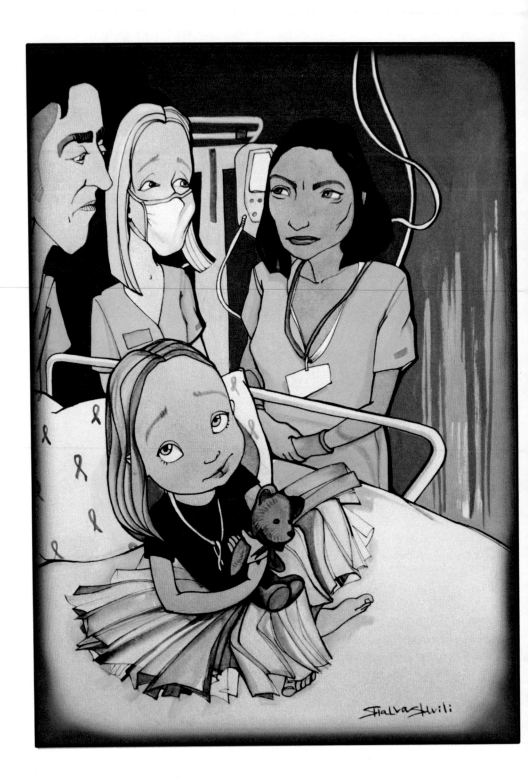

She took me to the emergency room to see a doctor. She was a very nice doctor but I was still scared because there were so many doctors and nurses in the room. I had to have a blood test and the needles hurt. I didn't know what was happening but I knew I wanted to go home. I could tell my mom was scared but she kept telling me everything would be alright as she hugged me.

The doctors didn't know what was wrong because the tests came back normal so they sent me to a hospital just for children. I had to have more tests and I was even more scared. I still don't remember anything about what my body was doing but my mom told me I kept drooling and would start to stare.

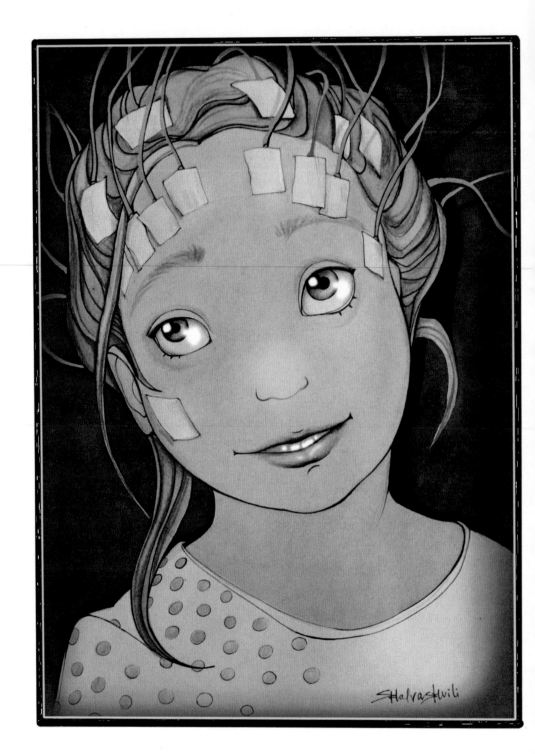

I remember a nice doctor putting little wires all over my head and lying down in a dimly lit room. I was told to close my eyes and lie still. I could see flashing lights every now and then and then they would stop. I had no idea what they were doing but was told it was to see what my brain was doing. It didn't take long and the man was funny and nice.

My mom said it was called an EEG which is also known as an electroencephalography that records brain activity along my scalp. It took a long time to clean off the gel since it was all over my head.

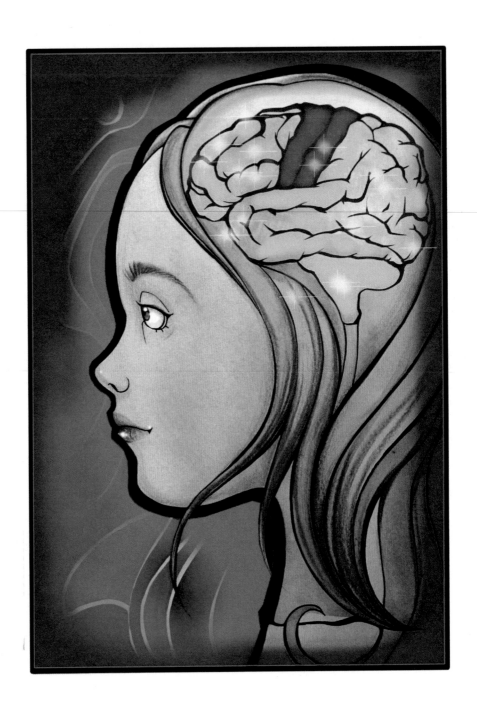

After a very long time, the doctors came in and told my mom that I had Benign Rolandic Epilepsy or BRE. Many children with BRE will eventually outgrow their epilepsy and I hope that I am one of them. They told my mom that epilepsy is a neurological condition and seizures are a sudden surge of electrical activity in the brain.

There are many different kinds of seizures and some people have a warning sign that happens before they will have one. Sometimes they might have a change in taste, sound, smell or might become scared or even have a headache. Some people might have a warning and some might not.

The doctors told my mom it was very important that I take my medicine twice a day at the same time every day. They also told my mom to keep a seizure diary to help the doctor the next time I had an appointment.

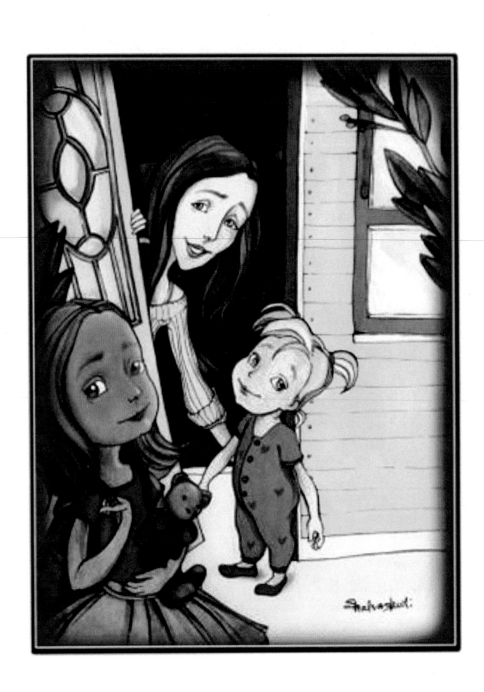

I was so relieved to be going home but I was still feeling funny. I almost felt like I was in a dream and wasn't really there. My mom brought me home and my sisters were happy to see me. I still kept feeling strange and I couldn't stop drooling. All I remember was it seemed like my brain was having a party and I was just watching.

I found that after my seizures, I would be confused and tired and just wanted to sleep. My mom told me that was normal and would tell me I should rest.

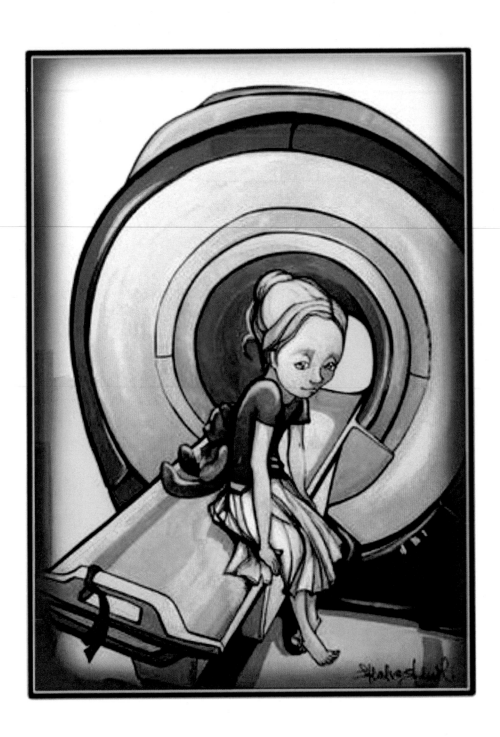

We went back to the hospital later and I was taken to a very weird machine called an MRI or magnetic resonance imaging to see what my brain was doing. It seemed like I was in the machine for a very long time and I was scared. My mom was not allowed to go with me but I had a very nice nurse who tried to make me happy. I don't remember much other than I did not hurt and I was so happy to see my mom again.

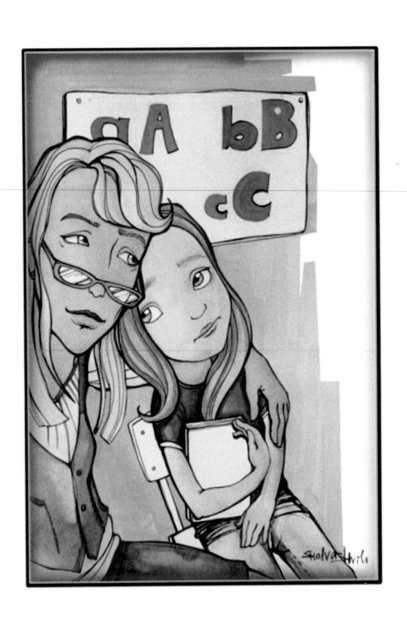

My epilepsy medicine was changed to Keppra because my mom said I was still drooling and was staring a lot. I also started kindergarten soon after being diagnosed with epilepsy.

I had a very nice teacher who tried to help me. I also started getting a lot of bad headaches. I would throw up and have to go home quite a bit. I don't remember having any seizures at school but I had a lot of headaches so my mom took me back to the doctor.

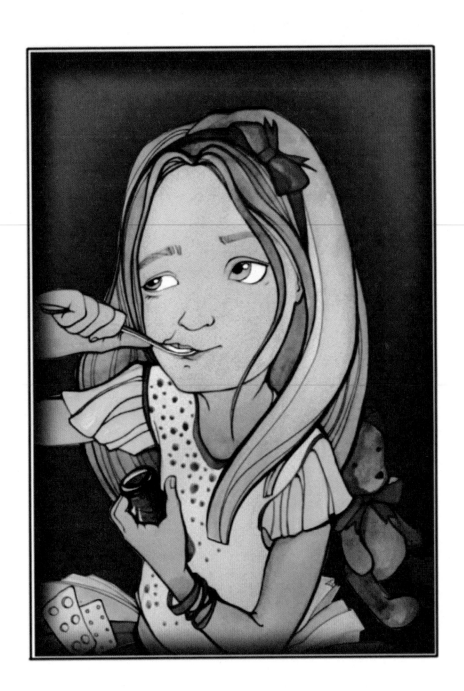

The doctor said I was having pediatric migraines and I had to now take another medicine that tasted bad. It tasted better than Keppra but it was still yucky. Every day before school, I had my medicine and again before I went to sleep. My mom always made sure I had my epilepsy medical alert bracelet on. I didn't like it because it bothered my skin but my mom said it was important in case I had a seizure and wasn't able to talk.

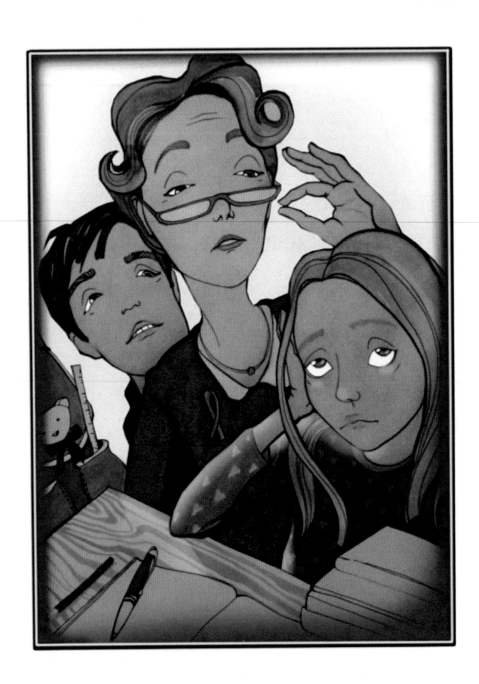

I had trouble at school because it seemed like everyone was faster than I was. I couldn't finish my work as fast as the other children and I always seemed to need help. This made me sad and I started to not like school. My favorite teacher, Mrs. Blount, was so good to me and this really helped. She tried to help me and took care of me like my mom would.

I had to repeat kindergarten because I was having problems finishing my work and keeping up with the other children. I was lucky because I was still not having any seizures and I know my mom was very happy.

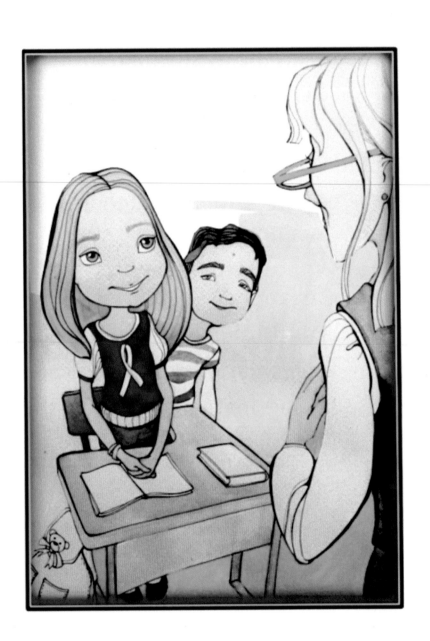

When I reached first grade, Mrs. Blount was my new teacher's assistant and I was so happy that I cried. I really liked Ms. Ayers and Mrs. Blount because they understood that I had epilepsy and needed a little more help. They tried everything to help me catch up and guess what? They did! I was finally beating time tests and getting good grades. I was very happy and started to like school again.

They understood that sometimes I might need some water, an extra snack or some rest. They knew that I might need a little extra time to finish my work or might need someone to explain something to me again. Epilepsy can affect children my mom said so that I wouldn't think it was anything to do with me. I know I am smart and that the epilepsy is just making some things a little harder.

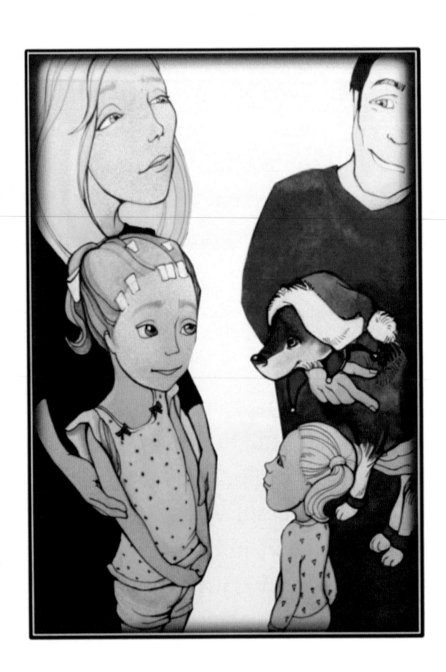

I had to go back to the hospital for an overnight video sleep study. This is where they hook you up to an EEG machine and monitor your brain activity for a period of time. My mom and I had so much fun because two groups of people brought Christmas presents and dogs for visits.

I received games and stuffed animals. My mom and I played games and made a play with our furry new friends that I still have in my toy boxes. We drew signs and my mom took pictures with her camera to send to my sisters who were at home. We laughed and laughed and had so much fun.

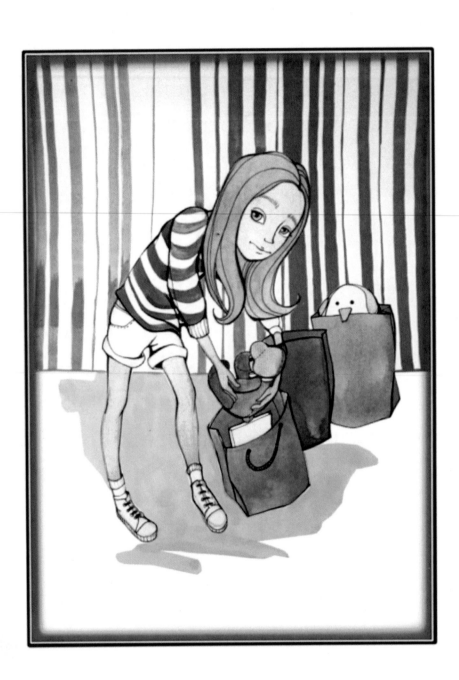

A little later, I decided that I wanted to do something nice for other children in the hospital so I came up with the idea to start delivering gift bags to children. My idea was called Angels4Epilepsy and we delivered our first gift bags full of toys, snacks and things to do to children who were in the hospital.

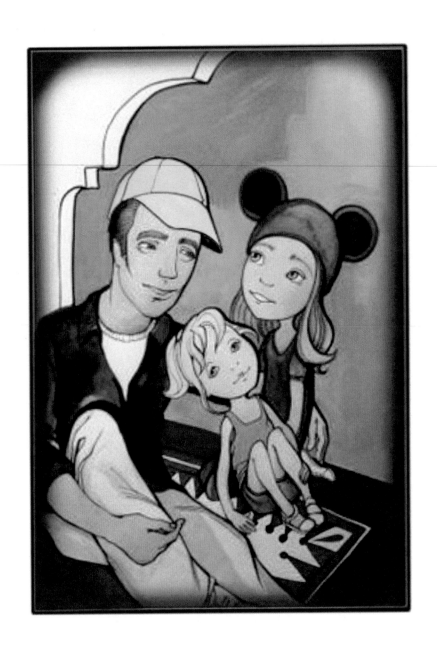

It has been three years since I was told I had epilepsy. I have been seizure free ever since and I still take my medicine every day. I don't like how it tastes but it's better than having a seizure.

I can ride a bike, ride a scooter, play on monkey bars, swim and do anything that other children can do. My mom just says I have to have a friend or an adult with me at all times and I can never take a bath by myself.

I can even go to Disney and have loads of fun!

I have epilepsy but it doesn't have me.

Made in the USA
Las Vegas, NV
18 March 2022

45921092R00019